GW00470614

Pocket Picture Guides

Oral Medicine

Pocket Picture Guides

Oral Medicine

Philip-John Lamey BSc BDS MB ChB DDS FDS RCPS

Senior Lecturer in Oral Medicine and Pathology,
Glasgow Dental Hospital and School,
Glasgow, UK

Michael A.O. Lewis BDS PhD FDS RCPS

Lecturer in Oral Medicine and Pathology,
Glasgow Dental Hospital and School,
Glasgow, UK

J.B. Lippincott Company • Philadelphia
Gower Medical Publishing • London • New York

Distributed in all countries except the
  USA & Canada by:
Harper & Row International,
10 East 53rd Street,
New York, NY. 10022, USA.

Distributed in the USA & Canada by:
J.B. Lippincott Company,
East Washington Square,
Philadelphia, PA. 19105, USA.

Library of Congress Catalog Number: 87-82127

British Library Cataloguing in Publication Data

Lamey, Philip-John
Oral medicine
1. Man. Mouth. Diagnosis
I. Title II. Lewis, Michael A.O.
616.3'1075

ISBN: 0-397-44575-X (Lippincott/Gower)

Project Editor: Michele Campbell
Design: Chris Inns

Printed in Hong Kong by South China Printing.
Set in Sabon and Frutiger by Dawkins Typesetters, London.

PREFACE

Oral medicine is that part of dentistry involved in the diagnosis and treatment of oral disease, which may be either localized or a manifestation of systemic illness. Generally, the speciality deals with disorders of the oral mucosa and of the salivary glands. However, the exact boundaries of oral medicine are ill defined and this book aims to illustrate the general areas of concern. Although neurological conditions such as facial pain are seen in oral medicine clinics, they are not covered here since they do not lend themselves to pictorial representation. Thus, this book does not provide a comprehensive coverage of oral medicine and should be supplemented by reading from standard texts. Treatment of the conditions illustrated is not discussed as this can vary between clinics and new approaches to management are continually being developed.

P-J. Lamey
M.A.O. Lewis
Glasgow

ACKNOWLEDGEMENTS

Most of the pictures in this book are taken from those held in the Department of Oral Medicine, Glasgow Dental Hospital and School, and the Department of Dental Surgery, Dundee Dental Hospital and School. We would like to express our special thanks to Professor D.M. Chisholm, Professor D.K. Mason, Dr J.G. Cowpe, Dr D. Stenhouse, Dr H.W. Noble, Miss E. Conor, Dr D.G. MacDonald, Dr M.M. Ferguson, Dr I.B. Watson, Dr P. Ebbesen and Mr W.J. Collins. Thanks are also due to Munksgaard for permission to publish Figures 62 and 63. Mrs I. McGuire kindly typed the initial manuscript.

CONTENTS

Preface   v

Acknowledgements   vi

Disorders of the teeth   1

Periodontal disease   10

Bone disorders   14

Disorders of the oral mucosa   18

Infections   26

Gastrointestinal and nutritional disorders   34

Haemopoeitic and endocrine disorders   38

Dermatological disorders   44

Disorders of the salivary glands   52

Tumours and localized lesions   58

Oral manifestations of drug therapy   68

Index   75

Disorders of the teeth

Abnormalities of tooth structure or morphology may be caused by genetic defects, drug therapy and a large number of systemic diseases. By far the commonest condition to affect tooth structure is dental caries.

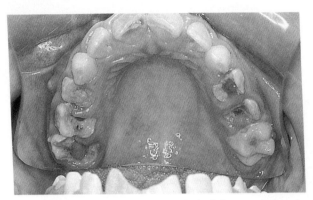

Fig. 1 A neglected mouth. Gross dental caries has led to extensive loss of tooth substance, particularly in the posterior quadrants. There is a chronic discharging sinus adjacent to the upper right molars and the crowns of the central incisors are fractured. Fortunately, this picture presents less frequently nowadays, as patients are more dentally aware and preventive measures, especially fluoride, are in widespread use.

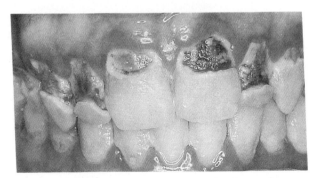

Fig. 2 Cervical caries. Extensive dental decay at this site is not common, but there are certain situations where it may occur. These include patients with xerostomia and those who ingest large amounts of drinks with a high sugar content. Some paediatric elixirs have a high concentration of sugar and have been responsible for producing a similar picture when given over extended periods.

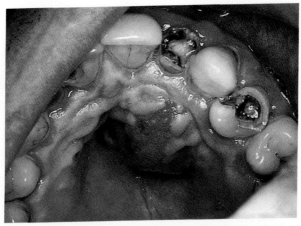

Fig. 3 Advanced dental caries. This has resulted in pulp death and subsequent formation of a dental abscess in the palate. Gross destruction of the lateral incisor tooth has occurred, leaving only the root visible.

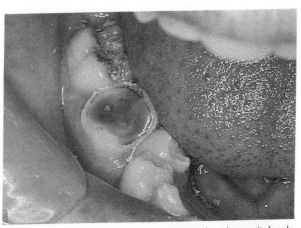

Fig. 4 Arrested dental caries. If the enamel walls of a carious cavity break down and expose the carious dentine to attrition, the surface becomes self-cleansing, with a reduction in carious activity. Although the dentine becomes stained, it stays hard and such teeth remain functional for many years.

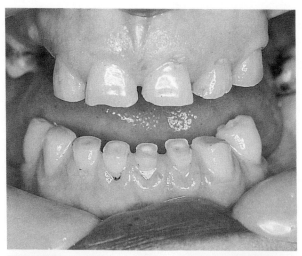

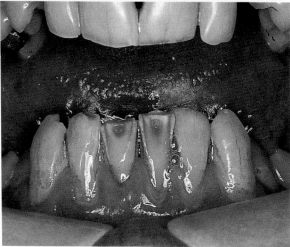

Fig. 5 Attrition. This is the slow process whereby loss of tooth substance is caused by heavy contact between opposing natural teeth. Where the teeth have an edge-to-edge relationship, the incisal edges are worn evenly (upper) and where there is a deep overbite, the labial surfaces of the lower incisors can be affected (lower).

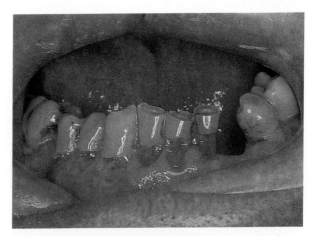

Fig. 6 Abrasion. Like attrition, abrasion is the wearing away of tooth substance by physical means; but whereas attrition is an endogenous process, abrasion is due to external factors. Severe notching in the cervical region of the teeth can result from an incorrect toothbrushing technique, as in this case.

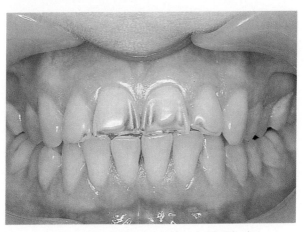

Fig. 7 Erosion. A localized high concentration of acid can lead to dissolution of the surface enamel. Smooth concave defects are seen on the labial surface of the upper incisors of this patient, who had the habit of sucking lemons.

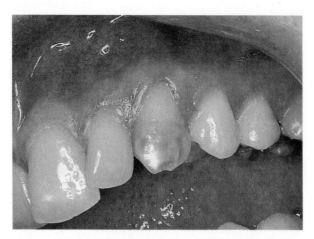

Fig. 8 Localized enamel hypoplasia (Turner's tooth). Periapical infection of a deciduous tooth can lead to brownish discoloration or pitting on the surface of the permanent successor. The extent of the hypoplasia depends on the severity and duration of infection during permanent tooth development.

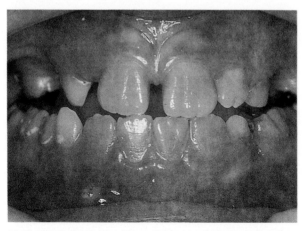

Fig. 9 Tetracycline staining. Tetracycline becomes incorporated into the teeth if given during periods of calcification. The position and extent of discoloration depend on the time and duration of therapy. The appearance of the affected teeth can be improved by crowns, veneers or bleaching techniques.

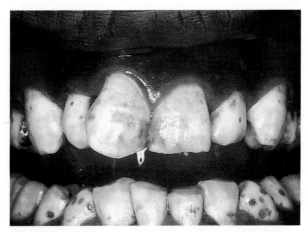

Fig. 10   Enamel fluorosis. If developing teeth are exposed to excessive fluoride levels in drinking water (>2ppm) the enamel formation is disturbed. The affected teeth show irregular areas of white opacity or brown staining. This condition is known as mottling.

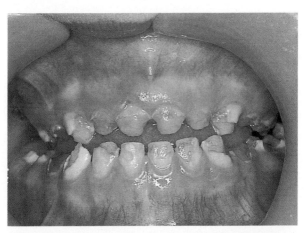

Fig. 11   Amelogenesis imperfecta. Enamel development is abnormal in this hereditary condition, which affects all the teeth in both dentitions. The teeth usually erupt with normal morphology, but the thin enamel wears rapidly. Surprisingly, they are not unduly susceptible to caries.

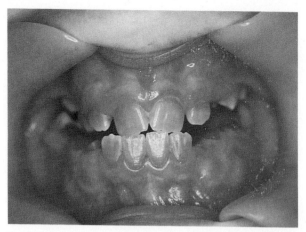

Fig. 12 Osteogenesis imperfecta. Several forms of this rare disease are recognized. It may be accompanied by blue sclerae and dentinogenesis imperfecta, in which the tooth form is essentially normal, but the teeth appear brown and abnormally translucent.

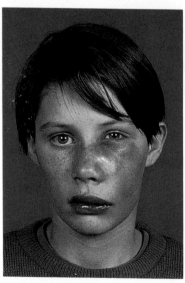

Fig. 13 Dentoalveolar abscess. Marked facial cellulitis with lip swelling and partial closure of the eye is characteristic of a periapical abscess affecting an upper anterior tooth.

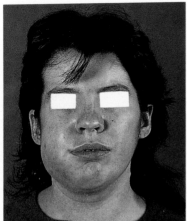

Fig. 14 Dentoalveolar abscess. This patient presented with swelling of the right cheek, tender cervical lymphadenopathy, trismus and pyrexia (left). Intraorally, a fluctuant erythematous swelling was present in the buccal sulcus (lower). Periapical infection had spread from the root apices of the upper first molar tooth.

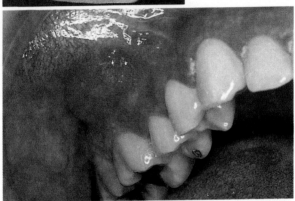

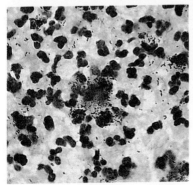

Fig. 15 Dentoalveolar abscess. This specimen was aspirated from an abscess. Such infections are commonly polymicrobial, containing a mixture of anaerobic Gram-positive cocci and Gram-negative bacilli (particularly *Bacteroides* species). Gram stain, ×1000.

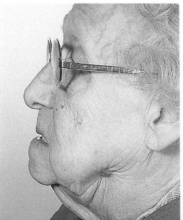

Fig. 16 Chronic facial sinus. Repeated infection over a period of years has resulted in marked tethering of the skin to the mandible (left). No tooth was evident clinically, but an orthopantomogram (lower) revealed an unerupted third molar as the source of infection.

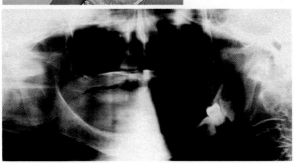

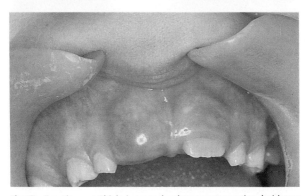

Fig. 17 Eruption cyst. This lesion may develop over an erupting deciduous or permanent tooth in children but does not significantly delay the process of eruption.

Periodontal disease

Gingivitis and periodontitis are pandemic and are the result of inadequate oral hygiene. Local and systemic factors may influence the severity of inflammation and the extent of periodontal destruction.

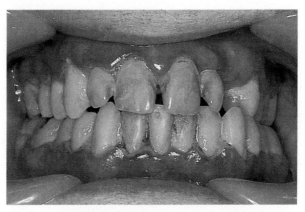

Fig. 18 Chronic gingivitis. Prolonged poor oral hygiene allows plaque to form on the teeth. The large number of microorganisms present in plaque provokes chronic inflammatory changes in the periodontal tissues. In this case the gingivae are red, oedematous and bleed easily on probing.

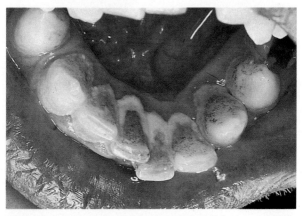

Fig. 19 Plaque and calculus. If plaque is not removed it becomes calcified to form calculus. Saliva constituents are thought to be involved in calculus formation, since heavier deposits are found on tooth surfaces adjacent to the duct outlets of the major salivary glands.

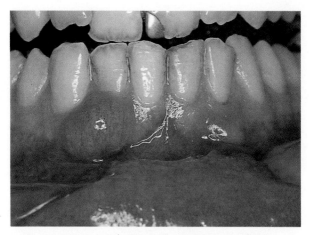

Fig. 20 Lateral periodontal abscess. A discrete fluctuant swelling is present on the gingival margin related to the right lateral incisor. The swelling was of sudden onset and was accompanied by localized throbbing pain. Distinction from a dentoalveolar abscess can be made by confirming the tooth's vitality. A similar abscess appears to be developing on the left lateral incisor.

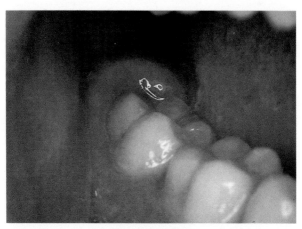

Fig. 21 Pericoronitis. Lower third molar teeth frequently have insufficient space to erupt fully into the mouth and infection occurs due to food and bacteria collecting under the flap of overlying mucosa (operculum). Opposing teeth may further traumatize the already swollen tissue. Patients complain of pain, swelling and difficulty in opening the mouth. In severe cases, lymphadenopathy and pyrexia are also present.

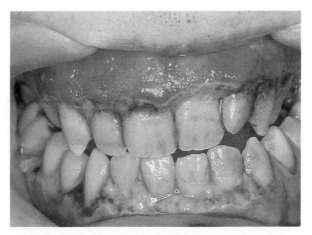

Fig. 22 Acute ulcerative gingivitis (Vincent's infection). This painful condition is of rapid onset and affects the gingival margins. Punched-out ulcers with surrounding erythema develop, leading to loss of the interdental papillae. Smears of affected areas show a mixed infection of fusobacteria and spirochaetes.

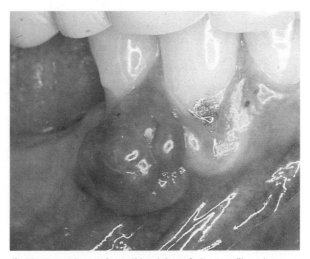

Fig. 23 Pyogenic granuloma. This painless soft-tissue swelling arises most frequently on the gingival margin and consists of vascular granulation tissue. The deep-red colour is due to its rich blood supply and the surface may bleed spontaneously or after minimal trauma. Apart from local irritation, the aetiology is not well understood.

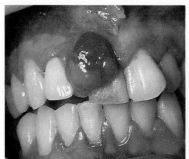

Fig. 24 Pregnancy epulis. This exophytic growth is clinically and histologically identical to pyogenic granuloma. The name has arisen because the lesion often develops during pregnancy. In some cases, spontaneous regression occurs after childbirth.

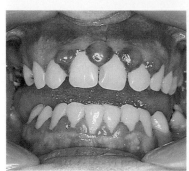

Fig. 25 Pregnancy gingivitis. The hormonal changes of pregnancy can result in gingival swelling and exaggerated inflammatory reactions to plaque. Classically, these changes are sharply limited to the interdental papillae.

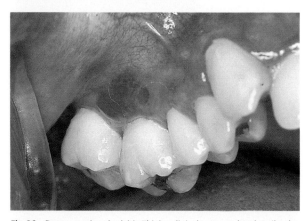

Fig. 26 Desquamative gingivitis. This is a clinical term used to describe the appearance of the gingivae in some patients with lichen planus, bullous pemphigoid or benign mucous membrane pemphigoid. Areas of the attached gingivae become thinned and have a fiery-red appearance.

Bone disorders

Although the jaws are infrequently affected by systemic disease of bone, structural defects due to traumatic fractures and development clefts are relatively common.

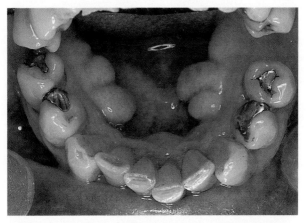

Fig. 27 Torus mandibularis. Bilateral bony swelling may develop on the lingual surface of the mandible in the premolar region. These exostoses appear between the first and third decades of life and consist of normal structured bone.

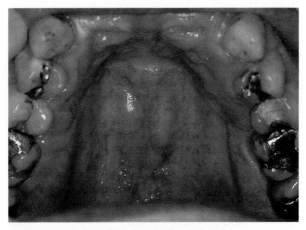

Fig. 28 Torus palatinus. This is the palatal equivalent of torus mandibularis. Both palatal and mandibular tori are asymptomatic but may complicate the provision of satisfactory dentures.

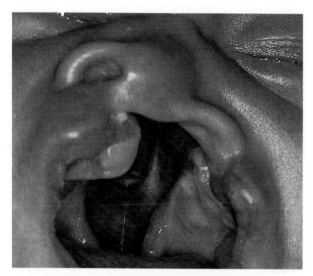

Fig. 29 Cleft lip and palate. A unilateral cleft of the lip with a complete cleft of the hard and soft palate. Wide separation of the lip cleft with alar displacement is apparent. The roof of the nasal passage can be seen through the large midline defect.

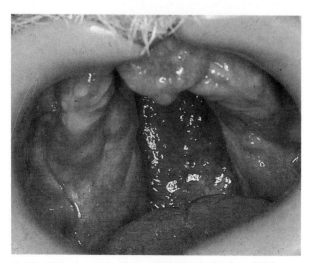

Fig. 30 Cleft palate. Cleft affecting the hard and soft palate which has not been repaired. Problems with speech and mastication can be improved by the provision of a suitable prosthesis.

15

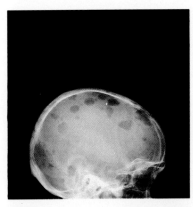

Fig. 31 Multiple myeloma. Lateral skull radiograph showing numerous discrete lytic lesions. The condition results from neoplastic proliferation of plasma cells. Amyloidosis is a common complication which may lead to macroglossia. Other intraoral features include bone pain, enlargement of the mandible or maxilla and localized bony exostoses.

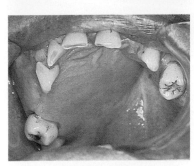

Fig. 32 Monostotic fibrous dysplasia. This condition is of unknown aetiology and several variants are recognized. Asymmetrical maxillary enlargement results in facial deformity and displacement of teeth. The overlying mucosa remains intact and appears healthy.

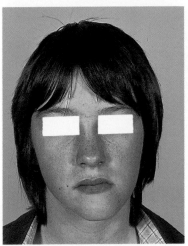

Fig. 33 Unilateral condylar hyperplasia. Condylar enlargement produces progressive elongation of the face and deviation of the chin away from the affected side. Although the enlarged condyle is easily palpated, joint function is usually normal.

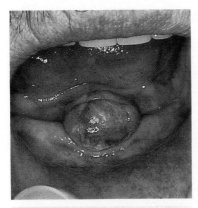

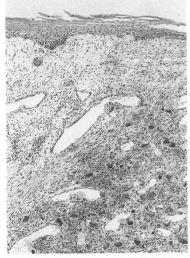

Fig. 34 Hyperparathyroidism. Primary hyperparathyroidism is uncommon but occasionally presents intraorally as cyst-like swellings, or epulides, of the jaw (upper). Radiographically, oral radiolucencies may be seen in the mandible, and affected areas show complete or partial loss of lamina dura around the teeth. Histological examination shows foci of osteoclasts (lower, H&E stain), which are indistinguishable from other giant cell granulomas of the jaws. Investigation of blood biochemistry is essential to confirm the diagnosis.

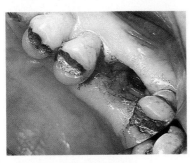

Fig. 35 Oroantral fistula. This is a direct communication between the maxillary antrum and oral cavity. It may be formed during extraction of upper premolar and molar teeth due to the proximity of the roots of these teeth to the maxillary antrum.

Disorders of the oral mucosa

A large number of conditions that affect the mouth do not fall specifically into areas covered by other sections of this book, therefore a variety of the more common developmental and acquired conditions are presented here.

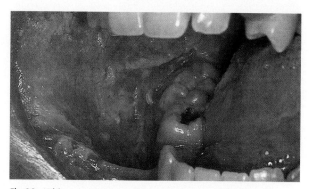

Fig. 36 White sponge naevus. This is a rare autosomal dominant condition, presenting in childhood as painless white folding of the oral mucosa. The lesion may be widespread, often involving the floor of the mouth, tongue and buccal mucosa. Any affected area should be biopsied to confirm the clinical diagnosis.

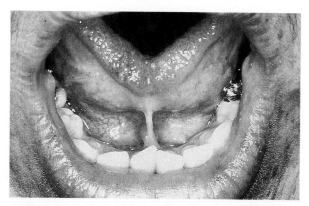

Fig. 37 Ankyloglossia (tongue-tie). This common developmental condition is the result of fusion between the tongue and the floor of the mouth. Tongue movements, particularly protrusion, are limited and in severe cases speech may be affected. Although present from birth, it is not uncommon for patients to present in adulthood, as the condition is frequently asymptomatic.

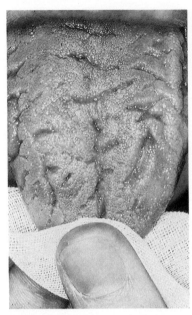

Fig. 38 Fissured tongue. In this condition, the fissures on the dorsal surface of the tongue are accentuated.

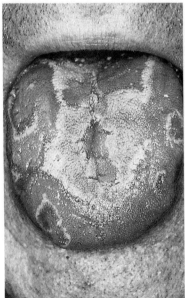

Fig. 39 Geographic tongue (erythema migrans). Irregular areas of papillary loss surrounded by a white border may develop on the dorsum of the tongue. The appearance characteristically changes with time, a feature which has led to the alternative name of benign migratory glossitis. Patients are usually asymptomatic, but some do complain of discomfort on eating.

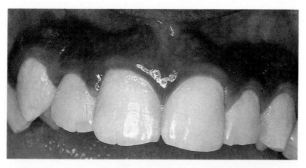

Fig. 40 Pigmentation. There is a wide variation in oral pigmentation amongst Caucasians and coloured races. In some people, extensive areas of the gingivae are deeply pigmented.

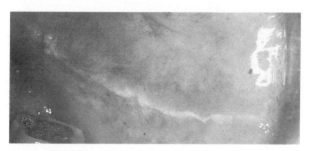

Fig. 41 Frictional keratosis. A discrete line of hyperkeratosis affecting the buccal mucosa can develop due to chronic trauma from the teeth during mastication. The line coincides with the plane of upper and lower teeth in occlusion.

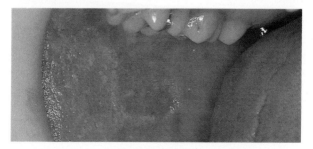

Fig. 42 Cheek biting. Habitual chewing of the buccal mucosa can be a nervous habit in some patients. The mucosa loses its smooth surface and assumes a rough texture, but this does not extend into the depth of the sulcus, nor beyond the posterior teeth.

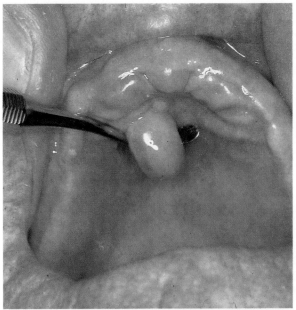

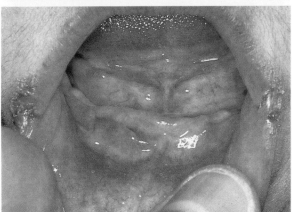

Fig. 43 Denture-induced hyperplasia. Chronic irritation from complete dentures can lead to hyperplastic changes in the oral mucosa. A solitary pedunculated lesion (leaf fibroma) may develop beneath the fitting surface of a complete upper denture (upper). In the lower arch, characteristic folding of the labial mucosa may be produced adjacent to the periphery of an ill fitting denture (lower). Note that this patient also has bilateral angular cheilitis.

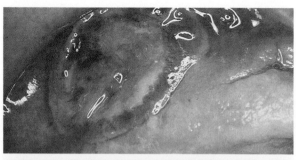

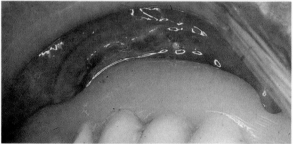

Fig. 44 Traumatic ulcer. A large ulcer with a fibrin base is present in the upper buccal sulcus (upper). It has arisen in an established area of denture-induced hyperplasia, and insertion of the upper denture clearly demonstrates the relationship of the ulcer to the labial flange (lower).

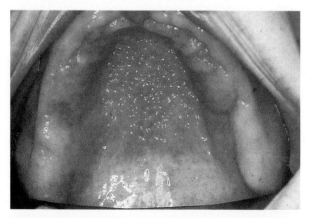

Fig. 45 Papillary hyperplasia. Numerous closely arranged papillary projections can be seen in the hard palate. This appearance is usually seen in denture wearers, but may also develop in patients with natural teeth.

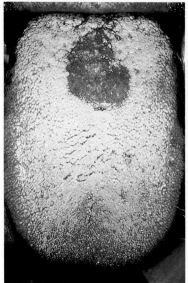

Fig. 46 Median rhomboid glossitis. A solitary diamond or rhomboid-shaped area of depapillation is apparent in the midline of the dorsum of the tongue, anterior to the circumvallate papillae. This condition has traditionally been considered as developmental in origin, however candidal infection has also been implicated.

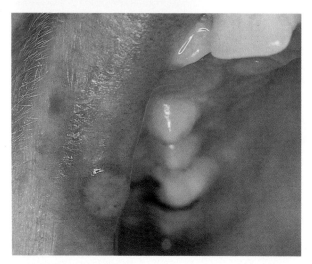

Fig. 47 Recurrent oral ulceration (minor aphthae). These small circular or oval ulcers have an erythematous border and can occur on any non-keratinized area of the oral mucosa. The ulcers are painful but heal in 4-14 days without scarring. Almost 1 in 5 of the population suffer from these ulcers at some time in their life, usually in adolescence or early adulthood.

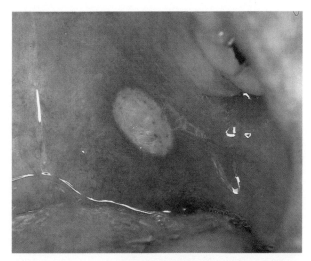

Fig. 48 Recurrent oral ulceration (major aphthae). In this less common form of aphthae, the ulcers are larger and take longer to heal. They have a tendency to affect the posterior region of the mouth, involving both keratinized and non-keratinized surfaces. Healing is slow (2-10 weeks) and may leave a residual scar.

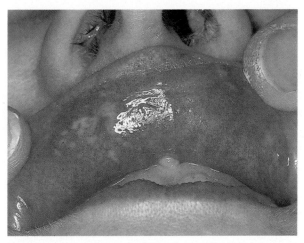

Fig. 49 Recurrent oral ulceration (herpetiform aphthae). This is the rarest form of aphthae and is characterized by numerous discrete ulcers, which coalesce to form large irregular lesions. The term 'herpetiform' is purely descriptive and does not imply a viral aetiology.

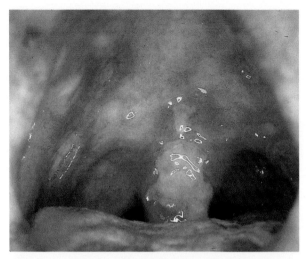

Fig. 50 Behçet's syndrome. This condition is characterized by severe ulceration of the palate, uvula and faucial region and resembles major aphthae. The diagnosis of Behçet's syndrome is made when recurrent genital ulceration or uveitis is also present.

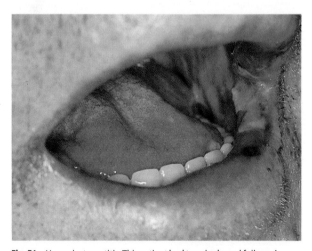

Fig. 51 Uraemic stomatitis. This patient had terminal renal failure. A pseudomembrane consisting of a viscous exudate was present on the erythematous buccal mucosa. The tongue was coated and ulceration had developed on the lateral margin. A heavy growth of *Candida albicans* was cultured from an oral rinse.

Infections

Caries and periodontal disease are the commonest of all infections. This section covers a number of specific infections of the oral mucosa and some oral manifestations of generalized infection. An underlying systemic disease may predispose to infection of unusual severity or duration.

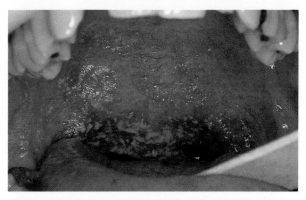

Fig. 52 Acute pseudomembranous candidiasis (thrush). Soft, creamy-yellow patches are present on the soft palate due to proliferation of *Candida albicans*. This presentation is not uncommon in patients on steroid inhaler therapy, particularly when they are also receiving broad-spectrum antibiotics.

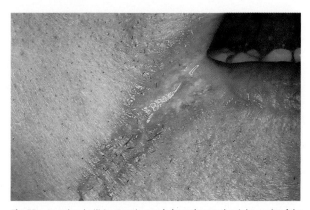

Fig. 53 Angular cheilitis. Crusting and ulceration at the right angle of the mouth, from which *Candida albicans* and *Staphylococcus aureus* were isolated. Intraoral candidiasis and haematological deficiency may be predisposing factors.

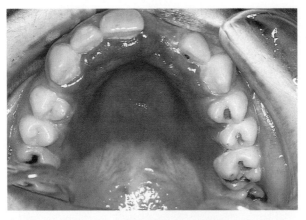

Fig. 54 Chronic atrophic candidiasis. The mucosa underlying this upper partial denture is erythematous and sharply demarcated from the adjacent healthy tissues. *Candida albicans* was isolated from both the denture-fitting surface and the inflamed mucosa. Continual denture wearing or poor denture hygiene creates an environment which favours candidal proliferation.

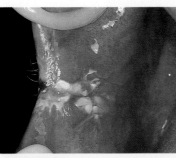

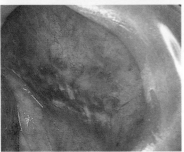

Fig. 55 Chronic hyperplastic candidasis (candidal leukoplakia). Chronic colonization of the oral mucosa by candidal species can lead to changes in the epithelium. In these two patients, firm white plaques of irregular thickness and outline are seen affecting the inner aspect of the angle of the mouth (upper) and the buccal mucosa (lower). The potential for malignant transformation in these lesions is well recognized.

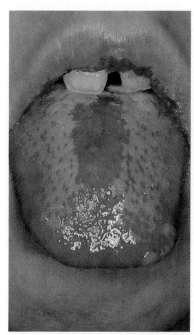

Fig. 56 Primary herpetic gingivostomatitis. This common infection of sudden onset is caused by *Herpes simplex* and usually occurs in childhood. Patients exhibit extensive oral ulceration, lip crusting, a furred tongue and are often pyrexial.

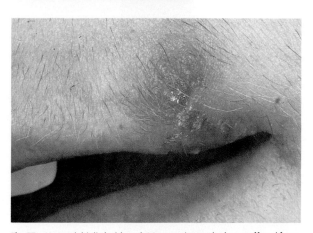

Fig. 57 Herpes labialis (cold sore). Many patients who have suffered from a primary herpetic infection are subsequently affected by recurrent herpes labialis. The vesicles rupture early to produce crusted ulcers which heal without scarring. Stress, fevers, local irritation, menstruation and exposure to sunlight are thought to lead to reactivation of the latent virus.

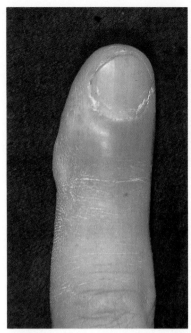

Fig. 58 Herpetic whitlow. This acute infection developed on a dentist's finger due to inoculation of *Herpes simplex* via a skin abrasion. The source of the virus was saliva from an infected patient. The condition is extremely painful and can be slow to resolve.

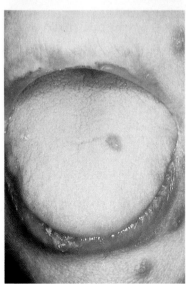

Fig. 59 Chickenpox (varicella). The characteristic vesicles of this viral infection are usually limited to the skin, but occasionally the oral mucosa is also affected.

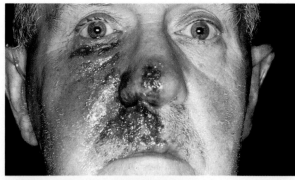

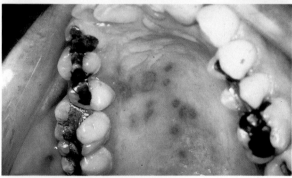

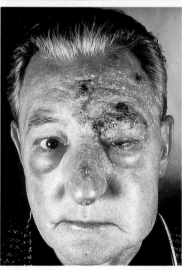

Fig. 60 Herpes zoster. This condition is the result of reactivation of varicella-zoster virus, acquired during a previous episode of chickenpox. The virus affects one or more branches of the trigeminal nerve unilaterally and severe localized pain may precede the development of vesicles. In these patients, the areas supplied by the maxillary (upper and middle) and ophthalmic (lower) divisions are shown.

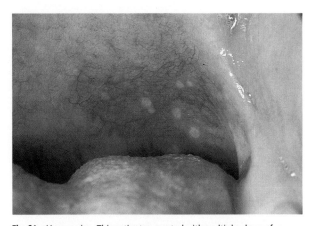

Fig. 61 Herpangina. This patient presented with multiple ulcers of varying size and a diffuse erythema affecting the soft palate and faucial region. The clinical manifestations of herpangina are of short duration and are comparatively mild. Different strains of Coxsackievirus (Group A) can lead to recurrent attacks.

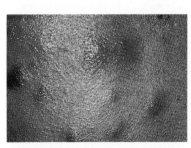

Fig. 62 Kaposi's sarcoma. Well demarcated macules are present on the skin of the cheek. This endothelial cell tumour can be a presenting feature of acquired immune deficiency syndrome.

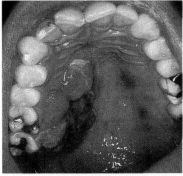

Fig. 63 Acquired immune deficiency syndrome. Kaposi's sarcoma has developed in the palate of this homosexual with AIDS. The tumour usually presents as a red/blue or purple patch. Other oral manifestations of AIDS include hairy leukoplakia, candidiasis and viral infections.

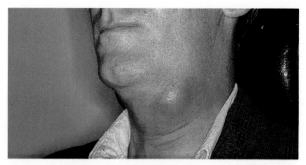

Fig. 64 Cervicofacial actinomycosis. This patient presented with a chronic firm localized swelling in the neck, which was slightly tender on palpation. The overlying skin had a dusky-red appearance. *Actinomyces israelii*, present in the patient's saliva, had gained entry to the subcutaneous tissues following extraction of a tooth. The pus drained from the lesion was seen to contain many characteristic sulphur granules.

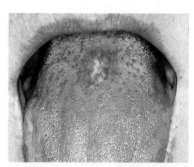

Fig. 65 Tuberculosis. A large indurated stellate ulcer is present on the dorsum of the tongue. This is a rare complication of open pulmonary tuberculosis with infected sputum.

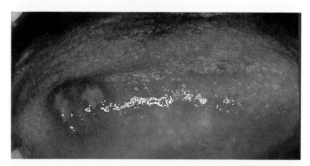

Fig. 66 Primary syphilis. Primary chancre of the tongue has developed following orogenital sexual contact with an infected partner. *Treponema pallidum* was demonstrated in exudate from the ulcers.

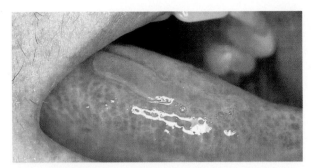

Fig. 67 Secondary syphilis. A flat painless ulcer with a grey membranous covering is present on the lateral border of the tongue. This is the so-called snail-track ulcer which, like the primary lesion, is highly infectious. Coincidentally, this patient also had lichen planus.

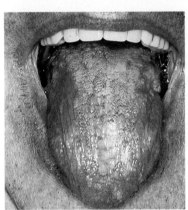

Fig. 68 Syphilitic leukoplakia. Leukoplakia on the dorsal surface of the tongue may occur in patients with tertiary syphilis. This condition can undergo transformation to squamous cell carcinoma.

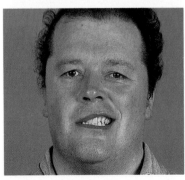

Fig. 69 Bell's palsy. This lower motor neurone disorder affects the facial nerve. The paralysis on the affected side leads to drooping of the corner of the mouth on smiling and inability to close the eye or wrinkle the forehead. An association with viral infection has been recognized in some patients.

33

Gastrointestinal and nutritional disorders

Oral lesions occur in a number of gastrointestinal diseases. Some may be directly attributable to the primary disease, but others are secondary lesions that arise due to malabsorption.

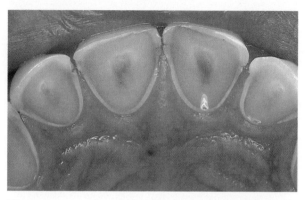

Fig. 70 Gastro-oesophageal reflux. Chronic regurgitation of gastric acid can produce erosion of the teeth, particularly the palatal surfaces of the upper anteriors. In the absence of functional pathology, this finding may be the first indication of a psychiatric or emotional disorder in which vomiting is self-induced.

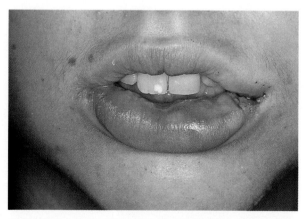

Fig. 71 Crohn's disease. The oral manifestations of this condition include irregular swelling of the lower lip, angular cheilitis and folded thickening of the buccal mucosa. The swelling is mainly due to lymphoedema. Biopsy of oral and intestinal lesions will reveal non-caseating granulomata.

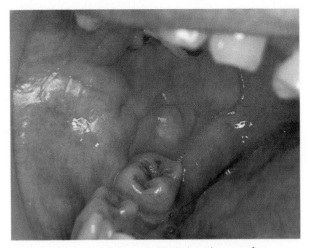

Fig. 72 Orofacial granulomatosis (OFG). The buccal mucosa often appears oedematous and biopsy down to muscle will demonstrate lymphatic dilatation and non-caseating granulomata. OFG appears to be a localized variant of Crohn's disease, in which patients are sensitive to foodstuffs, flavourings, dyes or preservatives.

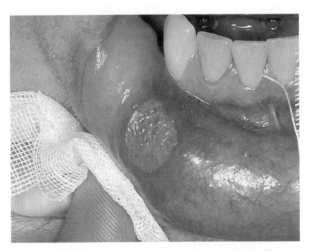

Fig. 73 Coeliac disease. This young woman, like many patients with coeliac disease, was folic acid deficient and initially presented with recurrent oral ulceration. The pathological basis for this condition is a sensitivity to dietary gluten, leading to abdominal pain and diarrhoea. Enteropathy is seen as villous atrophy on jejunal biopsy.

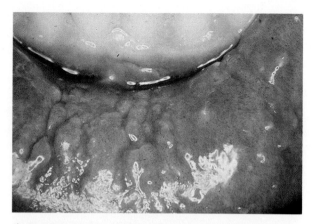

Fig. 74 Ulcerative colitis. This is an inflammatory bowel disorder of uncertain aetiology leading to gastrointestinal discomfort and malabsorption. Rarely, patients may develop irregular lesions of the lower lip (pyostomatitis vegetans) and oral ulcers which are identical to recurrent aphthae.

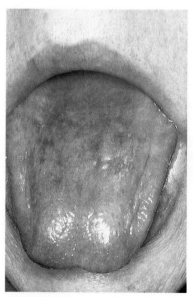

Fig. 75 Pernicious anaemia. Generalized papillary loss with mucosal atrophy affecting the dorsum of the tongue. This patient complained of soreness of the tongue, especially on eating. Haematological investigations revealed vitamin B_{12} deficiency and the diagnosis was confirmed by the Schilling test.

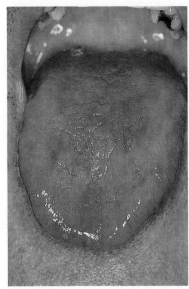

Fig. 76 Iron deficiency anaemia. In this case there is patchy loss of filiform and fungiform papillae on the dorsum of the tongue. This atrophic glossitis is less severe than that seen in patients with vitamin B_{12} or folic acid deficiency.

Haemopoeitic and endocrine disorders

Many abnormalities of the haemopoeitic and endocrine systems lead to changes in the health of the oral mucosa and associated structures. These changes may be the first sign of an underlying systemic disorder, as some endocrine and haemopoeitic conditions present with orofacial signs.

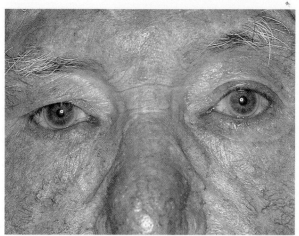

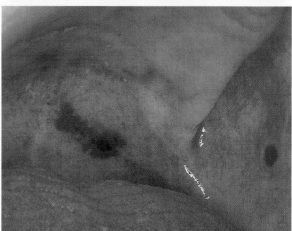

Fig. 77 Polycythemia rubra vera. The skin has a generalized cyanotic appearance and conjunctival suffusion is present as a result of capillary engorgement (upper). The oral mucosa is deep red with a bluish tinge and submucosal eccymoses are apparent (lower).

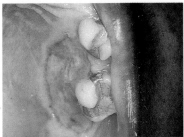

Fig. 78 Agranulocytosis. A large ulcer with minimal surrounding erythema is present in the hard palate. This condition requires early recognition, as oral and other infections are serious complications.

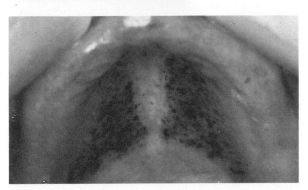

Fig. 79 Petechiae. Multiple pinpoint submucosal haemorrhages affecting a large area of the hard palate in a case of chronic idiopathic thrombocytopenic purpura.

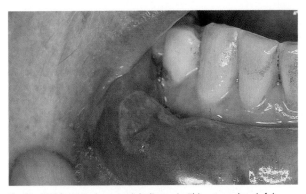

Fig. 80 Waldenström's macroglobulinaemia. This extremely painful, deep punched-out ulcer developed following accidental lip biting and took 4 weeks to resolve. The severity of the ulcer in relation to its trivial aetiology is highly suggestive of an underlying systemic illness.

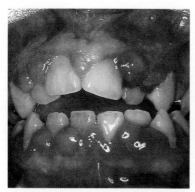

Fig. 81 Acute leukaemia. Any type of acute leukaemia, but particularly acute monocytic, may present with oral manifestations. In this patient the gingivae are hyperplastic, painful and bleed spontaneously. Such patients are susceptible to candidal, bacterial and viral infections.

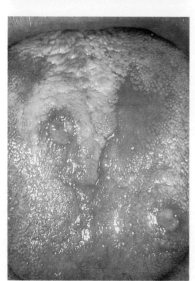

Fig. 82 Chronic leukaemia. This edentulous patient was receiving chemotherapy for chronic myeloid leukaemia. *Herpes simplex* was isolated from the ulcers, and *Candida albicans* from the coated areas on the dorsum of the tongue.

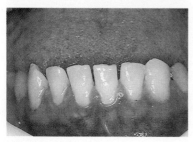

Fig. 83 Acromegaly. Enlargement of the mandible has led to spacing and forward tilting of the lower incisor teeth. Macroglossia has resulted in the lateral borders of the tongue having a scalloped appearance.

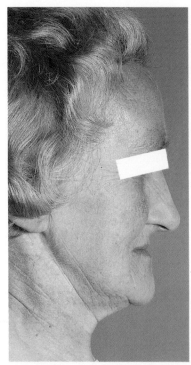

Fig. 84 Paget's disease (osteitis deformans). Facial profile showing frontal bossing (left). The patient complained of pain over her enlarged forehead. A lateral skull radiograph demonstrated the characteristic 'cotton-wool' appearance of bone (lower).

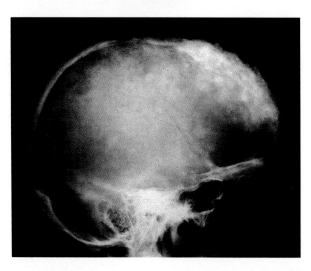

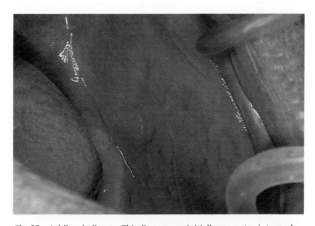

Fig. 85 Addison's disease. This disease may initially present as intraoral pigmentation, the colour varying from bluish-black to dark brown. The buccal mucosa, tongue, gingivae and lips can be affected. Tests of adrenocortical function are required for the final diagnosis.

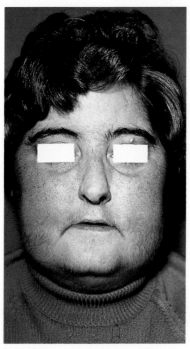

Fig. 86 Cushing's syndrome. This patient shows the typical moon face and hirsutism resulting from long-term, high-dose corticosteroid therapy. Persistent angular cheilitis and oral candidal infection were additional complications.

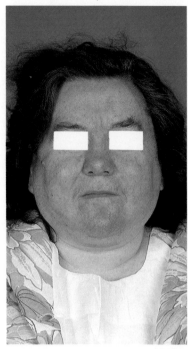

Fig. 87 Diabetes mellitus. Bilateral painless parotid gland enlargement in a patient with diabetes mellitus. This condition is known as sialosis and is a recognized, but rare, accompaniment to diabetes.

Dermatological disorders

It is not surprising that many cutaneous disorders have oral manifestations, given the similarity between the structure of the oral mucous membrane and that of the skin. Although many of these conditions remain asymptomatic, despite extensive mucosal involvement, some can produce severe symptoms.

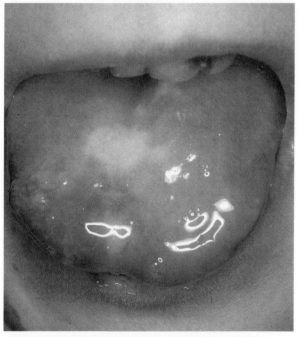

Fig. 88 Epidermolysis bullosa. Oral involvement can occur in the dystrophic form of this rare dermatological disease. Painful bullae may develop on any part of the oral mucosa and when the dorsum of the tongue is involved, as in this case, papillae are lost. Affected areas heal with scarring, which can lead to restricted tongue movements and limited mouth opening.

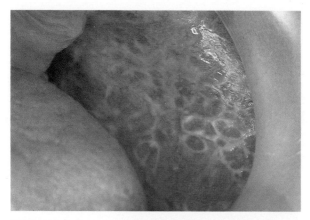

Fig. 89 Lichen planus. This is a chronic mucocutaneous condition and several oral changes are recognized clinically. The reticular form is seen here, presenting as discrete, painless, white striae affecting the buccal mucosa.

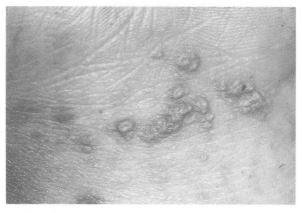

Fig. 90 Lichen planus. Classically, itchy, flat-topped, bluish-red papules with an overlying white network (Wickham's striae) occur at the wrist, but may also affect the flexor surfaces of the forearm and leg.

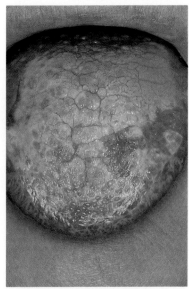

Fig. 91 Lichen planus. The plaque, or homogeneous type, is seen here on the dorsum of the tongue. The chronic and adherent nature of the lesions differentiates this condition from acute pseudomembranous candidiasis.

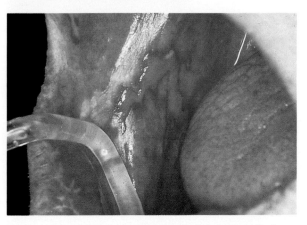

Fig. 92 Lichen planus. Irregular ulcers of erosive lichen planus affecting the buccal mucosa. The ulcers were painful, particularly on eating.

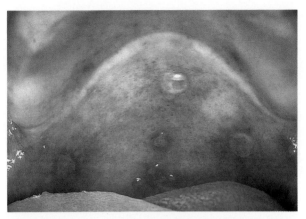

Fig. 93 Benign mucous membrane pemphigoid. In this bullous disorder, patients rarely present with intact bullae as they rupture at an early stage; it is more common to see areas of irregular oral ulceration.

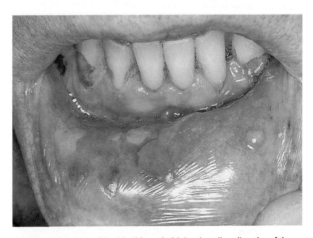

Fig. 94 Bullous pemphigoid. Although this is primarily a disorder of the skin, some patients later develop oral lesions identical to those of benign mucous membrane pemphigoid. In this case small multiple bullae, the majority of which have ruptured, developed beneath the labial mucosa.

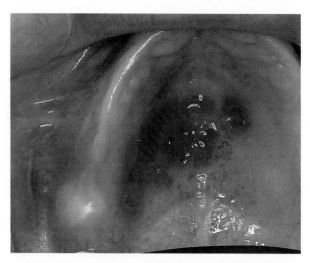

Fig. 95 Pemphigus vulgaris. This serious condition can affect any area of the oral mucosa and lesions often precede skin involvement. The painful intraepithelial bullae rupture early to leave irregular ulcers covered with a blood-tinged exudate.

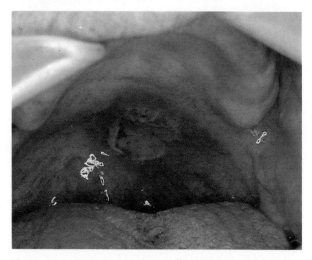

Fig. 96 Angina bullosa haemorrhagica. A large ulcer surrounded by a wide area of erythema is present in the soft palate. The patient reported that a large blood-filled blister developed whilst eating. It resolved within 5 days and left no scar. At present this condition is poorly understood.

48

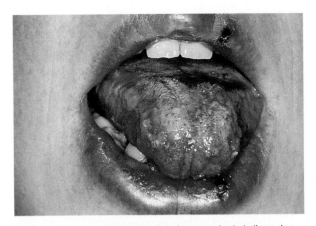

Fig. 97 Erythema multiforme. The clinical presentation is similar to that of primary herpetic gingivostomatitis but usually occurs in an older age group. The most striking features are swollen blood-crusted lips and widespread oral ulceration. The aetiology is unknown, however viral infections and a variety of drugs have been known to precipitate the condition. Erythematous skin lesions on the hands or feet may be accompanying features. Severe cases with eye involvement are termed Stevens-Johnson syndrome.

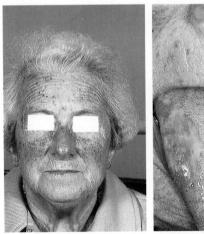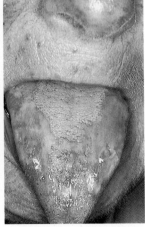

Fig. 98 Systemic lupus erythematosus (SLE). The facial appearance of a patient with long-standing untreated SLE (left). The butterfly rash is evident, although this can be a transient phenomenon. The dorsum of the tongue shows papillary loss and irregular atrophic areas (right).

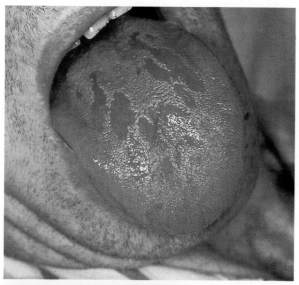

Fig. 99 Reiter's syndrome. The classical triad described by Reiter consisted of arthritis, urethritis and conjunctivitis. It is now recognized that the oral mucosa may also be involved. This tongue has areas of papillary loss and resembles geographical tongue, but the peripheral hyperkeratosis is absent (upper). The oral lesions are painless and resolve spontaneously. Genital manifestations take the form of a balanitis with a urethritis (left).

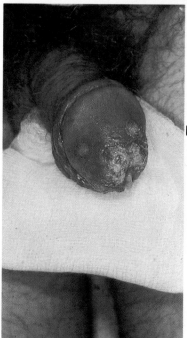

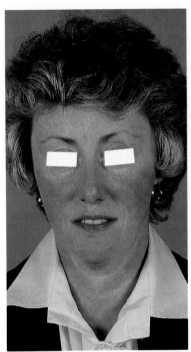

Fig. 100 Scleroderma. This is a chronic generalized sclerosis affecting the skin and other body systems. Involvement of the facial tissues causes immobility, pinching of the nose, limited mouth opening and involuntary exposure of the teeth.

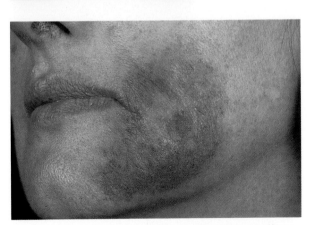

Fig. 101 Dermatitis artefacta. An erythematous skin lesion caused by a self-inflicted thermal burn. The patient will rarely admit how the lesion was produced, as an underlying emotional instability is usually present. Psychiatric assessment avoids inappropriate investigations and treatment.

Disorders of the salivary glands

Oral health is dependent upon normal function of the major and minor salivary glands. Reduced salivary secretion leads to a dry mouth, which in turn predisposes to oral infection and increased periodontal disease and caries activity.

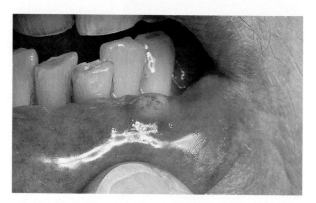

Fig. 102 Mucocele. Minor trauma to the duct outlets of the minor salivary glands can lead to extravasation of saliva into the surrounding connective tissue. The resultant small cysts are common on the lower lip, have a bluish appearance and are painless. Spontaneous discharge occasionally occurs but without treatment, recurrence is likely.

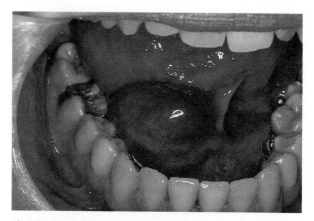

Fig. 103 Ranula. This large sublingual swelling is a form of mucocele associated with the ducts of the sublingual and submandibular glands. The bluish appearance is the result of accumulation of saliva. Although usually painless, it may interfere with swallowing, mastication and speech.

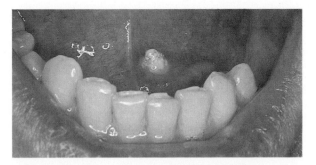

Fig. 104 Submandibular salivary calculus (sialolith). This patient complained of painful submandibular swelling occurring at mealtimes. A calculus, which had been enlarging within the submandibular duct for some time, eventually became lodged at the submandibular orifice, causing duct obstruction. The tip of the sialolith is evident clinically and palpation revealed a calcified mass extending along the duct.

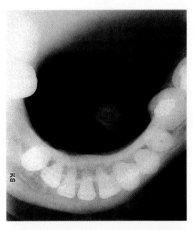

Fig. 105 Sialolith. Mandibular anterior occlusal radiograph showing a large sialolith at the anterior end of the submandibular duct. The sialolith had reached a surprisingly large size before signs of gland obstruction or infection supervened.

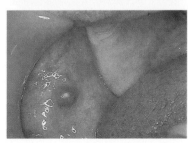

Fig. 106 Parotid calculus (sialolith). Compared to submandibular gland calculi, parotid calculi are uncommon but may cause gland obstruction due to blockage at the parotid orifice.

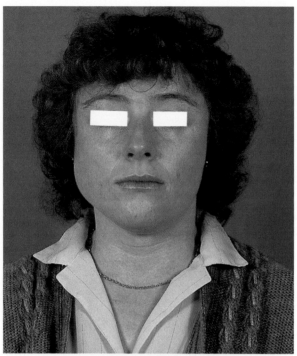
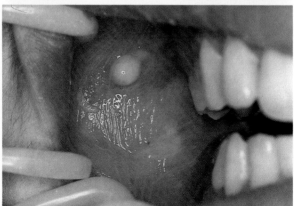

Fig. 107 Acute parotitis. This patient has a tender swelling of the right parotid gland (upper), and pus is present at the gland orifice (lower). In all such cases, once the acute infection has resolved with antibiotic treatment, a sialogram should be performed to exclude local gland abnormalities.

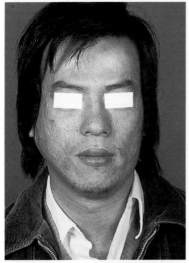

Fig. 108 Mumps (epidemic parotitis). This acute paramyxovirus infection has a predilection for salivary glands, particularly the parotids, and may be unilateral, as seen here, or bilateral. The condition usually occurs in childhood but if it affects adult males, orchitis can develop.

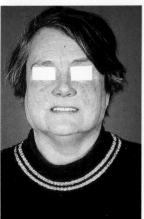 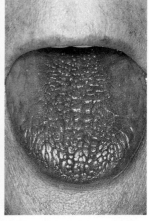

Fig. 109 Secondary Sjögren's syndrome. This inflammatory disorder of exocrine glands can be diagnosed when the patient has a connective tissue disorder (usually rheumatoid arthritis) and dryness of the eyes or mouth. Bilateral parotid gland enlargement is found in approximately 15% of these patients (left) and lacrimal gland function should be assessed by performing a Schirmer test. Assessment of keratoconjunctivitis requires a slit lamp examination. Intraorally, the mucosa is dry and atrophic due to reduced salivary flow rates, and in some patients the tongue has a lobulated or cobblestone appearance (right).

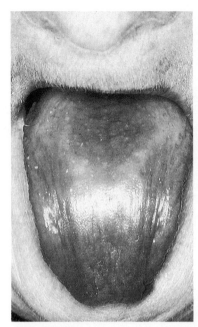

Fig. 110 Xerostomia (dry mouth). Long-standing reduced salivary gland function leads to generalized mucosal atrophy, which is particularly evident on the dorsum of the tongue. Diminished production of saliva may be due to disease of the glands or may be a side effect of drug therapy.

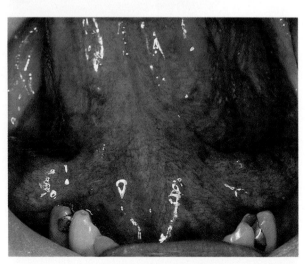

Fig. 111 Sarcoidosis. Bilateral sublingual gland enlargement in a case of generalized sarcoidosis. This condition is an uncommon, but recognized, cause of painful salivary gland enlargement.

56

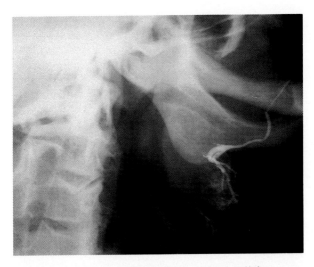

Fig. 112 Sialogram. Lateral oblique radiograph of a normal left submandibular salivary gland. Sialography is used to assess gland architecture. In this case, the curvature of the submandibular duct around the posterior border of mylohyoid is clearly seen, along with the normal branching pattern within the gland.

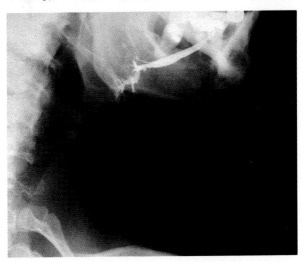

Fig. 113 Sialogram. This demonstrates narrowing of the submandibular duct just anterior to the gland and loss of normal structure. The patient had chronic submandibular sialadenitis.

Tumours and localized lesions

The vast majority of tumours that occur in the mouth are benign conditions, such as fibrous overgrowths. However, since intraoral carcinoma is not uncommon, it is essential that it is detected as early as possible. Unfortunately, oral cancer is often painless in the early stages and an extensive tumour may develop before it is noticed by the patient. During an oral examination the entire oral mucosa should be examined carefully and any suspicious lesion biopsied.

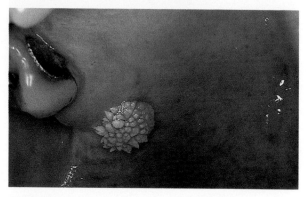

Fig. 114 Squamous cell papilloma. This lesion is benign and can affect any part of the oral mucosa. Typically, it is a pedunculated exophytic growth with numerous projections, producing a cauliflower-like surface.

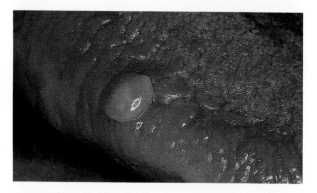

Fig. 115 Fibroepithelial polyp. Chronic minor irritation is believed to be involved in the development of these painless nodules, which often appear on the tongue and labial mucosa. The covering epithelium is characteristically smooth.

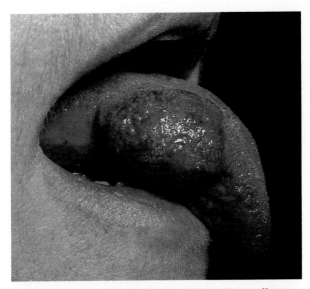

Fig. 116 Haemangioma. This developmental abnormality can affect any part of the oral cavity and is usually noticed at birth or in early childhood. Patients rarely have symptoms, although trauma can result in bleeding and ulceration with secondary infection.

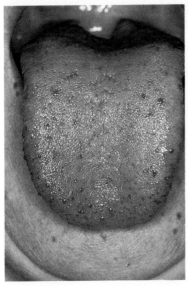

Fig. 117 Hereditary haemorrhagic telangiectasia (Rendu-Osler-Weber syndrome). Multiple angiomatous areas affect the skin and mucous membranes. Although present from birth, the lesions appear to increase in prominence in later life.

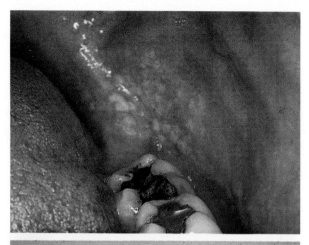

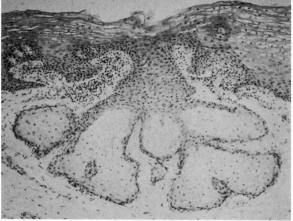

Fig. 118 Fordyce's spots. These are ectopic sebaceous glands without associated hair follicles. They appear as small, yellowish spots affecting the buccal and labial mucosae, often bilaterally (upper). Histologically, they consist of a discrete collection of sebaceous gland lobules with ducts opening onto the oral mucosa (lower). H & E stain.

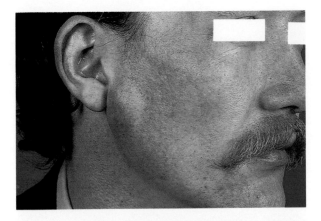

Fig. 119 Sebaceous cyst. A localized firm swelling over the right masseter region. Palpation revealed that the lesion was attached to overlying skin, which ruled out the provisional diagnosis of a parotid gland swelling.

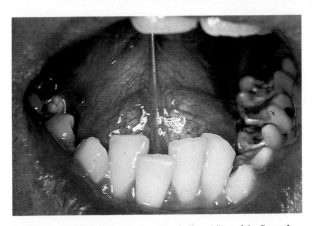

Fig. 120 Dermoid cyst. This raised swelling in the midline of the floor of the mouth is causing elevation of the tongue and difficulty with speech. The cyst is filled with keratin and sebaceous material and is soft on palpation.

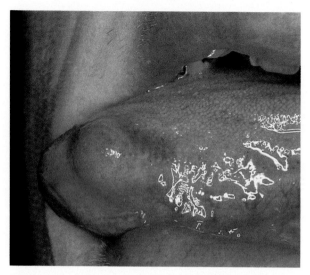

Fig. 121 Lipoma. These benign tumours of adipose tissue are rarely found in the oral cavity but when they do occur, they present as soft, round swellings in the tongue or cheek. The overlying mucosa has a normal appearance.

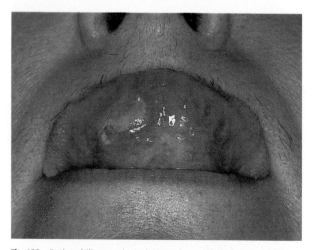

Fig. 122 Eosinophilic granuloma (traumatic granuloma). An irregular, well demarcated ulcer with a fibrin base can be seen on the ventral surface of the tongue. Although this rare condition may clinically resemble carcinoma, it is benign, self-limiting and heals without scarring.

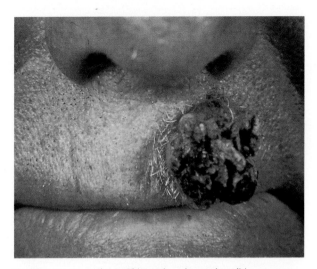

Fig. 123 Keratoacanthoma. This poorly understood condition occurs on exposed skin sites and can cause diagnostic difficulty since it resembles, even histologically, squamous cell carcinoma. The exophytic growth develops over a period of 4-8 weeks, persists for a similar period and then undergoes spontaneous regression.

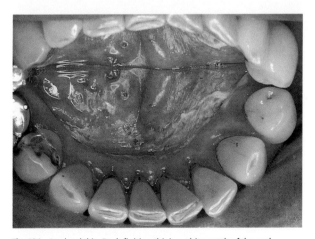

Fig. 124 Leukoplakia. By definition this is a white patch of the oral mucosa which cannot be rubbed off and is not attributable to any known cause. Lesions can be extensive and involve any area of oral mucosa. Biopsy is essential, as a proportion of leukoplakias undergo malignant transformation.

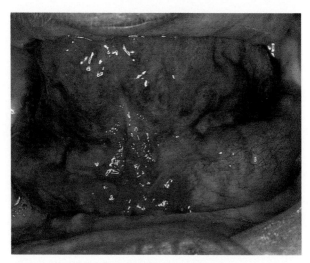

Fig. 125 Erythroplakia. A homogeneous red area of oral mucosa in the floor of the mouth. Erythroplakia has a high incidence of malignant transformation and is regarded as a precancerous condition.

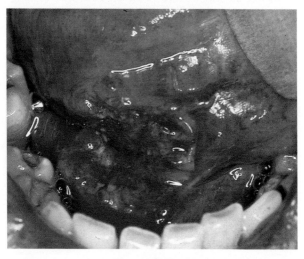

Fig. 126 Squamous cell carcinoma. This is by far the most common malignant tumour of the oral cavity and usually presents as a painless ulcer. The ulcer has raised borders and is firm on palpation. The intraoral sites most frequently affected are the floor of the mouth and the lateral border of the tongue.

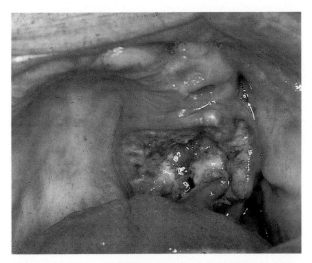

Fig. 127 Squamous cell carcinoma. A large deep ulcer with overhanging margins can be seen on the left palatal ridge. Metastatic spread to cervical lymph nodes had already occurred.

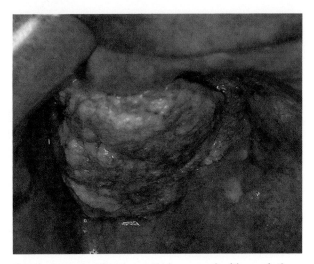

Fig. 128 Squamous cell carcinoma. This is an example of the exophytic type, seen here arising from the palatal alveolar ridge. The lesion was painless and had gradually increased in size over the preceding months. The patient presented only when the swelling prevented him from wearing his upper denture.

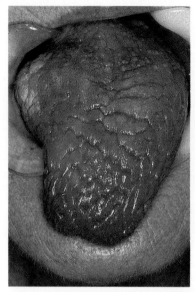

Fig. 129 Hypoglossal nerve palsy. A deeply invasive undifferentiated squamous cell carcinoma on the lateral border of the tongue has caused paralysis of the hypoglossal nerve. The loss of motor input results in the tongue deviating to the affected side on protrusion.

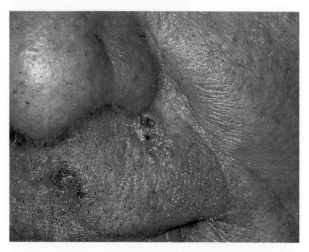

Fig. 130 Basal cell carcinoma. A small papule with central ulceration in the left alar region. If left untreated, progressive local tissue destruction is inevitable, although metastatic spread of this tumour is exceedingly rare.

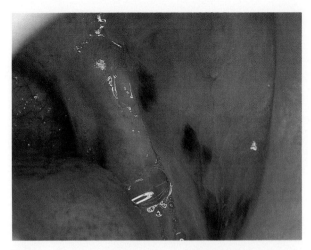

Fig. 131 Malignant melanoma. This tumour carries a high mortality rate, but fortunately it very rarely occurs intraorally. Any area of blue-black pigmentation must be treated seriously, especially if deepening in colour or increasing in size.

Oral manifestations of drug therapy

Conditions affecting the mouth are not uncommonly related to topical or systemic drug therapy and a variety of changes in the oral mucosa are recognized.

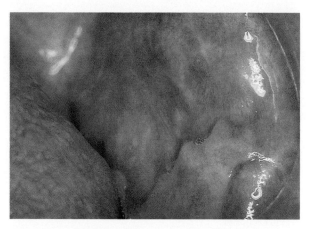

Fig. 132 Drug-induced oral ulceration. An occasional side effect of co-trimoxazole therapy is oral ulceration. In this case, a large irregular ulcer with widespread surrounding erythema has developed on the buccal mucosa. Withdrawal of the drug was followed by clinical resolution.

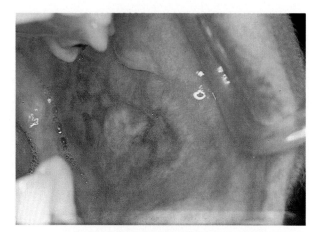

Fig. 133 Agranulocytosis. Multiple areas of ulceration with hyper-keratosis affecting the buccal mucosa. Haematological investigations confirmed the diagnosis of agranulocytosis induced by gold therapy.

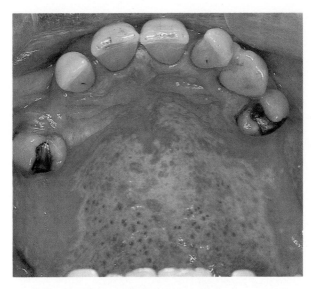

Fig. 134 Lichenoid reaction. This patient with maturity onset diabetes was managed by dietary control and glibenclamide. Shortly after the start of drug therapy, an extensive white patch developed in the palate which was histologically indistinguishable from lichen planus.

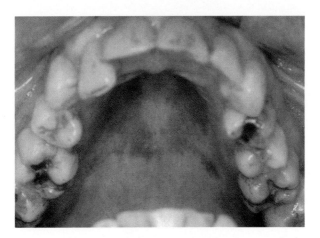

Fig. 135 Antimalarial pigmentation. Antimalarial drug therapy can lead to pigmentary changes affecting the skin and oral mucosa. In this case, the hard palate developed a slate-grey appearance after the patient had received several courses of amodiaquine.

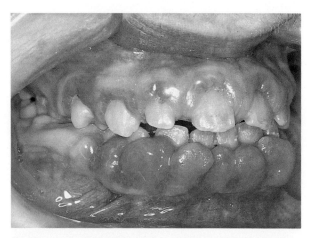

Fig. 136 Gingival hyperplasia. Painless enlargement of the gingivae is a well recognized side effect of the anticonvulsant drug, phenytoin. The swellings are firm, show little tendency to bleed and, in severe cases, may completely cover the teeth.

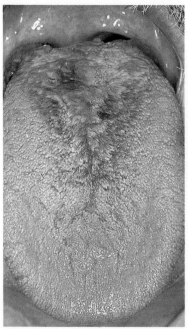

Fig. 137 Hairy tongue. Elongation of filiform papillae has led to a covering resembling hair on the dorsum of the tongue. A variety of drugs, particularly broad-spectrum antibiotics and oral iron preparations, can lead to this appearance.

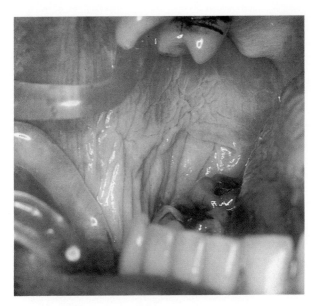

Fig. 138 Aspirin burn. The buccal mucosa and lateral surface of the tongue adjacent to two carious molar teeth appear white. Dissolution of aspirin tablets placed next to the painful teeth has resulted in a chemical burn of the surface mucosa.

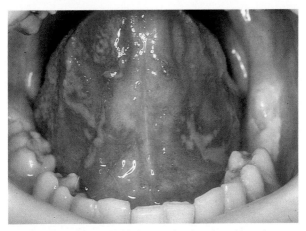

Fig. 139 Toothpaste sensitivity. This irregular ulceration with erythema affecting the ventral surface of tongue was due to sensitivity to the formaldehyde content of the patient's toothpaste.

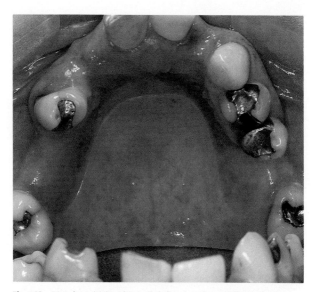

Fig. 140 Metal sensitivity. This well-defined erythema is limited to the area of mucosa covered by the chrome cobalt base of an upper partial denture. Repeated investigations for candidal infection were negative, but patch testing demonstrated a sensitivity to the denture base material.

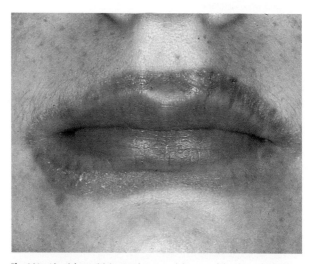

Fig. 141 Lipstick sensitivity. Erythema and dryness of the skin, which was thought to be due to the fluorescein component of the patient's lipstick.

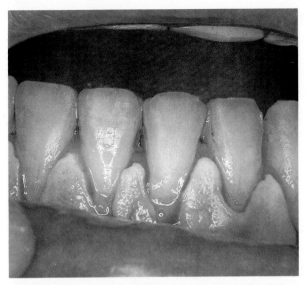

Fig. 142 Contact injury. This unusual reaction on the attached gingiva developed after dental treatment. A cotton-wool roll had been placed at this site for a prolonged period during the dental procedure.

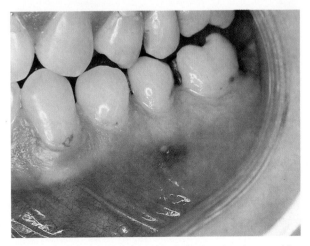

Fig. 143 Amalgam tattoo. Inadvertent introduction of amalgam particles beneath the oral mucosa can result in a persistent, localized area of blue pigmentation. This may occur during restorative procedures or at the time of tooth extraction.

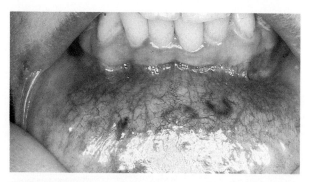

Fig. 144 Tattoo. In this clinical curiosity, the patient had attempted to tattoo the name Louise inside her lower lip.

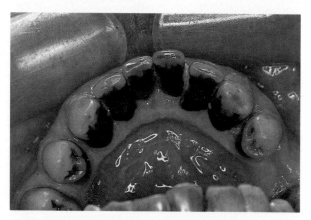

Fig. 145 Tobacco staining. The tars and resins present in tobacco smoke lead to varying degrees of staining of the tooth surfaces. The deposits do not cause structural damage to the teeth but do cause an aesthetic problem. Heavy tobacco smoking can give the tongue a black appearance.

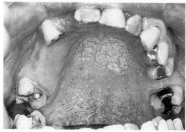

Fig. 146 Nicotinic stomatitis. Chronic irritation due to tobacco smoke and heat has led to hyperkeratosis in the palate. The minor salivary glands have become inflamed due to blockage of their ducts.

INDEX

Abscesses
  dentoalveolar 7,8
  palatal 2
  periodontal 11
Acquired immune deficiency
  syndrome (AIDS) 31
Acromegaly 40
Actinomyces israelii 32
Actinomycosis cervicofacial 32
Addison's disease 42
Agranulocytosis 39,68
Amalgam tattoo 73
Amelogenesis imperfecta 6
Amodiaquine 69
Amyloidosis 16
anaemia
  iron deficiency 37
  pernicious 36
Angina bullosa haemorrhagica 48
Ankyloglossia 18
Antibiotics, broad spectrum 70
Aphthae
  herpetiform 24
  major 24
  minor 23
Aspirin burn 71

Behcet's syndrome 25
Bell's palsy 33
Bone disorders 14–17

Calculus 10
  parotid 53
  submandibular 53
Candida albicans 25,26,27,40
Candidiasis
  acute pseudomembranous 26
  in AIDS 31
  chronic atrophic 27
  chronic hyperplastic 27
  Cushing's syndrome 42
Carcinoma
  basal cell 66
  intraoral 58
  squamous cell 33, 64,65,66

Caries *See* Dental caries
Chancre 32
Cheek biting 20
Cheilitis, angular 21,26,34,42
Chickenpox 29,30
Chrome cobalt, sensitivity to 72
Cleft lip 15
Cleft palate 15
Co-trimoxazole therapy 68
Coeliac disease 35
Cold sore 28
Colitis, ulcerative 36
Coxsackie virus 31
Crohn's disease 34, 35
Cushing's syndrome 42
Cutaneous disorders 44–51
Cysts
  dermoid 61
  sebaceous 61
  tooth eruption 9

Dental caries 1
  advanced 2
  arrested 2
  cervical 1
Dentinogenesis imperfecta 7
Dentures
  and candidiasis 27
  chrome cobalt, sensitivity to 72
  and hyperplasia 21
  and ulcers 22
Dermatitis artefacta 51
Dermatological disorders 44–51
Diabetes mellitus 43
  therapy 69
Drinks, sugar in 1
Drug therapy, oral manifestations
  68–71

Endocrine disorders 38,4002–3
Epidermolysis bullosa 44
Epulis
  in hyperparathyroidism 17
  pregnancy 13
Erythema migrans 19

Erythema multiforme 49
Erythroplakia 64

Facial nerve palsy 33
Facial sinus, chronic 9
Fibroma, leaf 21
Fistula, oroantral 17
Fluorosis, enamel 6
Folic acid deficiency 35
Fordyce's spots 60

Gastrointestinal diseases 34–6
Gastro-oesophageal reflux 34
Gingivae
   contact injury 73
   hyperplasia 70
   pigmentation 20,42
Gingivitis 10
   acute ulcerative 12
   desquamative 13
   pregnancy 13
Gingivostomatitis, primary
   herpetic 28
Glibenclamide 69
Glossitis
   benign migratory 19
   median rhomboid 23
Gold therapy 68
Granuloma
   eosinophilic 62
   pyogenic 12,13
   traumatic 62
Granulomatosis, orofacial 35

Haemangioma 59
Haemopoietic disorders 38–40
Herpangina 31
Herpes labialis 28
Herpes simplex 28,29,40
Herpes zoster 30
Hyperparathyroidism 17
Hyperplasia
   denture-induced 21–2
   drug induced 70
   papillary 22
Hypoglossal nerve palsy 66

Infections 26–33
Inhalers, steroid 26
Iron
   deficiency 37
   therapy 70

Kaposi's sarcoma 31
Keratoacanthoma 63
Keratosis, frictional 20

Leukaemia 40
Leukoplakia 63
   candidal 27
   hairy 31
   syphilitic 33
Lichen planus 13,33,45,46
Lichenoid reaction 69
Lip
   cleft 15
   lesions 36
   swelling 34
Lipoma 62
Lipstick sensitivity 72
Lymphoedema 34

Macroglobulinaemia,
   Waldenström's 39
Macroglossia 16,40
Malabsorption 36
Malaria, drug therapy 69
Mandible
   enlargement 40
   unilateral condylar hyperplasia
      16
Maxilla, asymmetrical
enlargement 16
Melanoma, malignant 67
Metal sensitivity 72
Mucoceles 52
Mucosa, disorders of 18–25
Mumps 55
Myeloma, multiple 16

Naevus, white sponge 18
Nicotinic stomatitis 74
Nutritional disorders 35–7

Oroantral fistula 17
Orofacial granulomatosis (OFG) 35
Osteitis deformans 41
Osteogenesis imperfecta 7

Paget's disease 41
Palate
  abscess 2
  cleft 15
  hard
    agranulocytosis 39
    papillary hyperplasia 22
    petechiae 39
Papilloma, squamous cell 58
Parotid gland
  calculus 53
  enlargement 43,54–5
  infections 54–5
Pemphigoid
  benign mucous membrane
    13,47
  bullous 13,47
Pemphigus vulgaris 48
Pericoronitis 11
Periodontal disease 10–13
  abscess 11
Phenytoin 70
Pigmentation, oral 20
  Addison's disease 42
  malignant melanoma 67
Plaque 10
Polycythemia rubra vera 38
Polyp, fibroepithelial 58
Pregnancy
  epulis 13
  gingivitis 13
Pulp death 2
Purpura, thrombocytopenic 39
Pyostomatitis vegetans 36

Ranula 52
Reflux, gastro-oesophageal 34
Reiter's syndrome 50
Rendu-Osler-Weber syndrome 59

Saliva, diminished production 56
Salivary glands, disorders 52–7
Sarcoidosis 56
Sarcoma, Kaposi's 31
Schilling test 36
Schirmer test 55
Scleroderma 51
Sebaceous glands, Fordyce's
  spots 60
Sialogram 57
Sialolith 53
Sialosis 43
Sjögren's syndrome 55
Steroid inhalers 26
Stevens–Johnson syndrome 49
Stomatitis
  nicotinic 74
  uraemic 25
Sublingual gland, enlargement 56
Submandibular gland
  calculus 53
  sialogram 57
Sugar in drinks 1
Syphilis 32, 33
Systemic lupus erythematosus
  (SLE) 49

Tattoo 74
Teeth
  abrasion 4
  abscesses 7,8
  attrition 3
  caries 1–2
  disorders 1–9
  enamel
    abnormal development 6,7
    dissolution 4
    fluorosis 6
    hypoplasia 5
  erosion 4,34
  eruption cyst 9
  mottling 6
  tetracycline staining 5
  tobacco staining 74
  unerupted, infection from 9

Telangiectasia, hereditary
  haemorrhagic 59
Tetracycline staining of teeth 5
Thrombocytopenic purpura 39
Thrush 26
Tobacco
  smoke, irritation 74
  staining 74
Tongue
  cobblestone appearance 55
  fissured 19
  geographic 19
  hairy 70
  macroglossia 16, 40
  median rhomboid glossitis 23
  –tie 18
Toothpaste sensitivity 71
Torus mandibularis 14
Torus palatinus 14
Treponema pallidum 32
Tuberculosis 32
Tumours 58–67
Turner's tooth 5

Ulcerative colitis 36
Ulcers
  dentures and 22
  drug-induced 68
  herpangina 31
  herpetic 28
  recurrent 23–5,35
  snail-track 33
  syphilitic 32,33
  tubercular 32

Varicella 29,30
Vincent's infection 12
Vitamin B12 deficiency 36

Waldenström's
  macroglobulinaemia 39
Whitlow, herpetic 28
Wickham's striae 45

Xerostomia 56